Copyright 2023

All right reserved.No part of this book should be reproduced without express permission of the author.

Reproduction of all or any part of this book is punishable unders relevant law.

Table of Contents

PREVIEW

The word cerebrovascular is made up of two parts — "cerebro" which refers to the large part of the brain, and "vascular" which means arteries and veins. Together, the word cerebrovascular refers to blood flow in the brain. The term cerebrovascular disease includes all disorders in which an area of the brain is temporarily or permanently affected by ischemia or bleeding and one or more of the cerebral blood vessels are involved in the pathological process. Cerebrovascular disease includes stroke, carotid stenosis, vertebral stenosis and intracranial stenosis, aneurysms, and vascular malformations.

Restrictions in blood flow may occur from vessel narrowing (stenosis), clot formation (thrombosis), blockage (embolism) or blood vessel rupture (hemorrhage). Lack of sufficient blood flow (ischemia) affects brain tissue and may cause a stroke.

CEREBROVASCULAR DIET RECIPES

BREAKFAST

1. Cheesesteaks

Prep Time: 5 Minutes

Cook Time: 20 Minutes

Servings: 2

Ingredients

- 6 large eggs, divided
- 2 tablespoons milk
- 4 thick slices bread
- 1 (5 ounce) Sausage Patties
- 1 tablespoon olive oil
- 1 clove garlic, minced
- ½ red bell pepper, thinly sliced
- ½ green bell pepper, thinly sliced

- ½ small red onion, thinly sliced
- 2 slices provolone cheese
- Salt and pepper, to taste

Instructions

1. In medium bowl, whisk together 2 eggs and milk; dip bread into egg mixture until fully coated. Cook French toast on griddle or large skillet over medium heat until golden brown on both sides.
2. Cook sausage patties according to package instructions. Cut into strips.
3. In separate skillet, heat olive oil over medium heat. Add garlic, peppers and onions and saute until browned and tender.
4. Add cooked sausage strips to pepper and onion mixture; top with cheese and heat until cheese is melted.
5. Cook remaining eggs over easy, or as desired.
6. Assemble cheesesteaks by layering french toast with eggs, and pepper, sausage and cheese mixture. Season with salt & pepper and serve open-faced.

Prep Time: 15 Minutes

Cook Time: 1hrs 10 Minutes

Servings: 8

Ingredients

- 1 green onion, chopped
- 1 (16 ounce) package hash brown potatoes
- 2 cups shredded Cheddar cheese
- 6 large eggs, lightly beaten
- 1 cup milk
- 1 (2.64 ounce) package country gravy mix
- 1 pinch ground paprika, or to taste

Instructions

1. Preheat the oven to 325 degrees F (165 degrees C). Grease an 8x11-inch baking dish.
2. Cook and stir breakfast sausage in a skillet over medium heat until browned and crumbly, about 10 minutes; drain excess grease.

3. Mix green onion into the sausage and spread into the bottom of the prepared baking dish. Spread hash brown potatoes in a layer over top; sprinkle with Cheddar cheese.

4. Whisk eggs, milk, and gravy mix together in a bowl until smooth; pour over casserole. Season with paprika.

5. Bake in the preheated oven until a knife inserted into the center of the casserole comes out clean, about 1 hour. Let stand 10 minutes to firm up before serving.

Prep Time: 5 Minutes

Cook Time: 30 Minutes

Servings: 2

Ingredients

- 2 medium pork sausage patties
- 1 tomato
- 2 tablespoons butter, divided
- 2 slices bacon
- ¼ (16 ounce) package frozen hash browns, thawed
- 1 (6 ounce) package sliced fresh mushrooms
- 1 (15 ounce) can baked beans
- 1 large egg
- 2 slices bread
- salt and ground black pepper to taste
- 1 sprig fresh parsley, chopped

Instructions

1. Preheat the oven to 425 degrees F (220 degrees C).

2. Brown the sausages on all sides in a frying pan over medium heat for 5 minutes. Transfer to a baking dish.

3. Bake the sausages in the preheated oven for 10 minutes.

4. Score a cross into the bottom of the tomato and place, cross-side up, in the baking dish with the sausages.

5. Bake the sausages and the tomato for 10 minutes. Turn off the oven, but do not remove the sausages and tomato.

6. Meanwhile, in the frying pan used to brown the sausages, melt 1 tablespoon of butter and fry the bacon, hash browns, and the mushrooms over high heat until the mushrooms have softened, the bacon begins to crisp, and the hash browns turn golden, about 7 minutes. Transfer to the oven to keep warm.

7. Pour beans in a small saucepan and cook, stirring frequently, over medium heat until heated through.

8. Crack egg into a skillet over medium heat. Cook until outer edges become opaque, about 1 minute. Cover, reduce heat to low, and cook until whites are completely set, about 4 minutes.

9. Toast bread and spread remaining butter over.

10. Bring together the sausages, hash browns, bacon, beans, tomato, mushrooms, fried egg, and toast on a

warm serving plate. Season with salt and pepper, garnish with parsley, and serve immediately.

3. Breakfast Burrito

Prep Time: 15 Minutes

Cook Time: 30 Minutes

Servings: 4

Ingredients

- 2 pounds beef skirt steak, cut into thin strips
- 2 tablespoons carne asada seasoning
- 1 tablespoon garlic powder
- 1 tablespoon vegetable oil
- ½ sweet onion, diced
- 1 red bell pepper, seeded and chopped
- 1 jalapeno pepper, seeded and diced
- (14.5 ounce) can Hunt's Diced Tomatoes, drained
- cups frozen diced potatoes
- Salt and pepper to taste
- tablespoons butter, divided
- 6 eggs, whisked
- 2 cups shredded Mexican cheese blend
- (12 inch) flour tortillas

Instruction

1   Place beef slices in a mixing bowl. Sprinkle with asada seasoning and garlic powder; toss in bowl to evenly coat. Let marinade 5 minutes.

2   Heat oil in a large, deep skillet over medium-high heat. Place beef strips in skillet and cook and stir until browned. Stir in bell pepper, onions, and jalapeno pepper. Add tomatoes and potatoes. Cook mixture until potatoes are tender, 5 to 8 minutes. Season with salt and pepper. Transfer mixture to a bowl.

3   Melt 1 tablespoon butter in the same skillet. Add the eggs, stirring occasionally, until eggs are scrambled and set. Transfer the beef mixture back to skillet. Cook and stir until warmed through, about 2 minutes. Melt the remaining 2 tablespoons butter in a small dish in microwave.

4   Divide shredded cheese among tortillas; divide beef and veggie mixture and place on the cheese. Fold in sides of tortilla and roll up. Brush with melted butter and place folded side down in pan to brown; flip and brown on top side. Burrito should be warmed though.

Prep Time: 25 Minutes

Cook Time: 30 Minutes

Servings: 4

Ingredients

- 1 Caulipower Pizza
- 1 teaspoon olive oil
- slices turkey bacon
- ¼ cup chopped onion
- ¼ cup chopped red bell pepper
- 1 cup chopped fresh spinach
- 1 clove garlic, minced
- ½ cup egg whites
- ¼ cup shredded Cheddar cheese
- 1 tablespoon chopped fresh basil (Optional)

Instructions

1   Preheat the oven to 425 degrees F (220 degrees C). Place pizza on a baking sheet.

2   Bake in the preheated oven for 13 to 15 minutes.

3   Meanwhile, heat olive oil in a frying pan. Saute bacon, onion, and bell pepper in the hot oil until tender, 8 to 10 minutes. Drain off any grease and return to the pan. Add chopped spinach and garlic; stir until spinach is wilted. Remove from the pan to a small bowl to let cool for a few minutes.

4   Remove pizza from oven. Leave oven on. Add egg whites to vegetable mixture; stir to combine.

5   Carefully top pizza with vegetable-egg mixture. Pour slowly so eggs don't run off the sides. Use a spoon to catch any drips and return to the top of the pizza.

6   Bake in the preheated oven for 10 minutes. Top with Cheddar cheese and bake for 5 minutes more. Remove from the oven and top with fresh basil.

Prep Time: 25 Minutes

Cook Time: 6hrs 10 Minutes

Servings: 8

Ingredients

- 12 large eggs
- 1 cup heavy cream (or half-and-half)
- 1 teaspoon onion powder
- 1 teaspoon salt
- ½ teaspoon black pepper
- ¼ teaspoon crushed red pepper flakes
- (20 ounce) package refrigerated hash brown potatoes
- ounces shredded Parmesan cheese, divided
- ounces shredded mozzarella cheese, divided
- 1 (5 ounce) Sausage Links, sliced into coins
- ½ cup chopped sun-dried tomatoes, divided
- ½ cup chopped fresh basil, divided

Instructions

1   Spray slow cooker with non-stick cooking spray.

2   In medium bowl combine eggs and cream; whisk until well combined. Sprinkle onion powder, salt and both peppers over egg mixture while whisking. Whisk until completely combined. Set aside.

3   In slow cooker, combine hash browns and about 1/2 of each of Parmesan cheese, mozzarella cheese, sausage, sun-dried tomatoes and basil. Using fingers, gently toss until combined. Pour egg mixture over top; if necessary use spatula to smooth out top.

4   Set aside about 1/2 of remaining mozzarella cheese (approximately 2 ounces). Sprinkle remaining ingredients over top of casserole. Cover slow cooker and cook for 6-8 hours on low or until center is cooked through. A thermometer inserted into center should read 160 degrees F.

5   Sprinkle casserole with remaining cheese, serve and enjoy!

Prep Time: 15 Minutes

Cook Time: 1hrs

Servings: 4

Ingredients

- 3 corn tortillas, cut into 1-inch pieces
- ½ cup chopped ham
- ½ cup diced tomatoes
- ½ cup salsa
- ¼ cup milk
- ¼ cup shredded sharp Cheddar cheese
- ¼ cup shredded jalapeno Jack cheese
- 2 tablespoons chopped fresh cilantro
- 2 medium green onions, sliced
- 3 large eggs
- ¾ cup milk
- Salt and freshly ground black pepper to taste
- ¼ cup crumbled cotija cheese

Instructions

1. Preheat the oven to 350 degrees F (175 degrees C). Grease a 5x7-inch glass dish.

2. Mix ham, tomatoes, salsa, 1/4 cup milk, Cheddar cheese, jalapeno Jack cheese, cilantro, and green onions.

3. Place half of the tortillas into the prepared baking dish and top with half of the ham mixture. Repeat layers. In another bowl, mix eggs, 3/4 cup milk, salt, and pepper. Pour over mixture in the baking dish.

4. Bake in the preheated oven until top starts to brown, 60 to 75 minutes. Remove from the oven and let sit for 10 minutes before cutting. Sprinkle with cotija cheese.

Prep Time: 30 Minutes

Cook Time: 15 Minutes

Total: 45 Minutes

Servings: 18

Ingredients

- 1 cup warm milk
- 1 egg, lightly beaten
- 1 egg yolk, beaten
- 3 cups bread flour
- ½ tablespoon salt
- 3 tablespoons butter
- ¼ cup white sugar
- 3 teaspoons bread machine yeast

Filling:

- 18 2 inch sausages, cut in 1/2
- (16 ounce) package frozen hash brown potatoes
- slices Cheddar cheese, quartered

Instructions

1   In the order suggested by the manufacturer, place milk, egg, egg yolk, bread flour, salt, butter, sugar and bread machine yeast in bread machine. Select Dough cycle, and press Start.

2   Preheat oven to 375 degrees F (190 degrees C). Lightly grease a large baking sheet.

3   On a lightly floured surface, punch down dough, and divide into 36 pieces. Roll pieces into balls. Arrange balls in a single layer on the prepared baking sheet, about 2 inches apart. Allow balls to rise 15 to 20 minutes.

4   Flatten balls, and make a depression in the center of each. Fill each with 1 piece of sausage, about 1 tablespoon hash browns, and 1 quarter slice of cheese.

5   Bake 15 to 18 minutes in the preheated oven, or until lightly browned.

Prep Time: 15 Minutes

Cook Time: 30 Minutes

Total: 45 Minutes

Servings: 8

Ingredients

- 2 (22.5 ounce) packages frozen hash brown
- 2 tablespoons butter
- large eggs, beaten
- ½ teaspoon kosher salt
- ¼ teaspoon ground black pepper
- (8 ounce) package shredded Cheddar cheese
- 10 slices cooked bacon, chopped
- teaspoons chopped fresh chives, or to taste

Instructions

1   Preheat the oven to 450 degrees F (230 degrees C).

2   Arrange 12 hash brown patties in a single layer on a rimmed baking sheet; it's okay if they overlap a bit. Reserve remaining patties for another use.

3   Cook in the preheated oven for 10 minutes.

4   Remove from the oven and use a spatula to press the edges of each hash brown together so they slightly stick together and fill the baking sheet. Return to the oven and cook until golden and crisp, about 15 more minutes.

5   While the hash browns are in the oven, melt butter in a medium nonstick skillet over medium heat. Add eggs, salt, and pepper and cook, stirring often, until very soft scrambled, 3 to 4 minutes; they will finish cooking in the oven.

6   Remove hash browns from the oven. Sprinkle with ¾ cup Cheddar cheese, then top evenly with scrambled eggs. Sprinkle bacon and remaining Cheddar over top. Return to the oven until cheese is melted, 3 to 5 more minutes.

7   Sprinkle with chives before cutting and serving.

Prep Time: 20 Minutes

Cook Time: 40 Minutes

Total: 60 Minutes

Servings: 8

Ingredients

- cooking spray
- (16 ounce) package bacon
- large eggs
- 1 cup milk
- ½ medium red bell pepper, chopped
- ½ medium yellow bell pepper, chopped
- ½ medium onion, chopped
- ¼ cup chopped fresh cilantro, or to taste
- Salt and ground black pepper to taste
- ½ cup croutons, or more to taste
- ½ cup shredded pepper Jack cheese, or more to taste
- ½ cup shredded Cheddar cheese, or more to taste
- ½ cup shredded Swiss cheese, or more to taste

Instructions

1. Preheat the oven to 350 degrees F (175 degrees C). Lightly spray a square baking pan with cooking spray.

2. Place bacon in a large skillet and cook over medium-high heat, turning occasionally, until evenly browned, about 10 minutes. Drain bacon slices on paper towels and chop when cool enough to handle.

3. Whisk eggs and milk together in a bowl. Mix in bell peppers, onion, cilantro, salt, and pepper.

4. Arrange croutons in the bottom of the prepared pan. Layer with chopped bacon, then pepper Jack, Cheddar, and Swiss cheeses. Pour the egg mixture over the top.

5. Bake in the preheated oven until set, 30 to 40 minutes. Remove from the oven and let sit for 20 minutes before serving.

Prep Time: 10 Minutes

Cook Time: 55 Minutes

Servings: 12

Ingredients

- 1 pound sliced bacon, diced
- 1 medium sweet onion, chopped
- large eggs, lightly beaten
- cups frozen shredded hash brown potatoes, thawed
- 2 cups shredded Cheddar cheese
- 1 ½ cups small curd cottage cheese
- 1 ¼ cups shredded Swiss cheese

Instructions

1   Preheat the oven to 350 degrees F (175 degrees C). Grease a 9x13-inch baking dish.

2   Heat a large skillet over medium-high heat; cook and stir bacon and onion until bacon is evenly browned, about 10 minutes. Drain.

3   Transfer bacon and onion to a large bowl. Stir in eggs, potatoes, Cheddar cheese, cottage cheese, and Swiss cheese. Pour mixture into the prepared baking dish.

4   Bake in the preheated oven until eggs are set and cheese is melted, 45 to 50 minutes. Let stand 10 minutes before cutting and serving.

LUNCH

Prep Time: 15 Minutes

Cook Time: 35 Minutes

Total: 50 Minutes

Servings: 6

Ingredients

- 2 tablespoons unsalted butter
- 2 cups chopped onions
- 1 ½ pounds fresh mushrooms, thickly sliced
- ½ teaspoons chopped fresh dill
- 1 tablespoon Hungarian sweet paprika
- tablespoon soy sauce
- 2cups low-sodium chicken broth
- 1 cup skim milk
- 3 tablespoons all-purpose flour
- ½ ripe tomato
- ½ Hungarian wax pepper
- 1 teaspoon salt

- ground black pepper to taste
- ½ cup light sour cream

Instructions

1. Melt the butter in a large pot over medium heat. Cook and stir the onions in the butter until fragrant, about 5 minutes. Add the mushrooms and continue cooking until the mushrooms are tender, about 5 minutes more. Stir the dill, paprika, soy sauce, and chicken broth into the mushroom mixture; reduce heat to low, cover, and simmer 15 minutes.

2. Whisk the milk and flour together in a small bowl. Stir the mixture into the soup. Add the tomato and Hungarian wax pepper. Return cover to the pot and simmer another 15 minutes, stirring occasionally. Season with salt and pepper. Mix the sour cream into the soup and continue cooking and stirring until the soup has thickened, 5 to 10 minutes more. Remove the Hungarian wax pepper and tomato and discard before serving the soup.

Prep Time: 20 Minutes

Cook Time: 15 Minutes

Servings: 8

Ingredients

- 1 sheet pastry dough for 9-inch tart
- ounces frozen chopped spinach, thawed and drained
- cups frozen hash brown potatoes, thawed
- 1 ½ cups shredded Gruyere cheese, divided
- large eggs, beaten
- ½ cup heavy cream
- 2 teaspoons everything bagel seasoning
- 3.dashes hot pepper sauce, or to taste

Instructions

1 Preheat the oven to 400 degrees F (200 degrees C). Cut a 9-inch circle of parchment paper.

2 Place pastry crust in a 9-inch quiche or pie pan, gently shaping and stretching to fit. Prick crust with a fork several times and place parchment circle over top.

Add pie weights or dried beans on top of parchment paper.

3   Set the pan on a baking sheet and place in the center of the preheated oven. Reduce heat to 375 degrees F (190 degrees C) and bake about 10 minutes. Remove to a wire rack and cool for about 5 minutes. Carefully remove pie weights or beans and parchment paper. Leave oven on.

4   While the crust is cooling, squeeze thawed spinach between several layers of paper towels, to remove most of the moisture. Set aside.

5   Add thawed potatoes to the cooled crust. Sprinkle 1 cup shredded Gruyere cheese on top.

6   Stir beaten eggs, cream, bagel seasoning, and hot pepper sauce in a large bowl until ingredients are fully incorporated. Stir in spinach, breaking up any clumps. Pour mixture over the cheese and potatoes. Sprinkle the remaining 1/2 cup Gruyere on top.

7   Place in the center of the oven and bake until eggs are set and a knife inserted into the middle comes out clean, 40 to 45 minutes. Remove from the oven and cool on a rack for 10 minutes. Serve warm

Prep Time: 10 Minutes

Cook Time: 45 Minutes

Servings: 4

Ingredients

- tablespoons olive oil
- 1 bunch green onions, chopped
- 2 (5 ounce) packages fresh baby spinach
- tablespoons water, divided
- 2 (3 ounce) packages ramen noodles (flavor packets discarded)
- large eggs
- ¾ cup garlic-and-herb spreadable cheese (such as Alouette
- ¼ teaspoon salt
- ¼ cup grated Parmesan cheese

Instructions

1   Preheat oven to 375 degrees F (190 degrees C).

2   Heat oil in a 10-inch ovenproof skillet (with lid) over medium heat. Cook green onions, stirring occasionally, until softened, about 2 minutes. Add 1 package spinach and 2 tablespoons water and cook, covered, until wilted, about 1 minute. Stir spinach with tongs, then add remaining package spinach and remaining tablespoon water. Cook, covered, stirring once or twice, until tender, about 2 minutes. Remove skillet from heat.

3   Meanwhile, bring a saucepan of salted water to a boil. Break each ramen noodle block into 4 pieces and cook, stirring occasionally, until just tender, about 3 minutes. Drain noodles in a colander and rinse under cold water. Toss noodles with spinach mixture in skillet and spread mixture evenly over bottom of pan.

4   Blend eggs, spreadable cheese, and salt in a blender until smooth. Pour egg mixture evenly over spinach mixture. Stir spinach mixture gently with a fork to allow egg mixture to flow underneath. Sprinkle top with Parmesan cheese.

5   Transfer skillet to oven and bake until puffed slightly and a toothpick inserted in center comes out clean, about 35 minutes. Cut into 4 wedges and serve from skillet.

Prep Time: 20 Minutes

Cook Time: 30 Minutes

Servings: 4

Ingredients

- (10 ounce) packages frozen chopped spinach
- matzo crackers
- eggs, beaten
- Salt and pepper to taste
- 1 pinch ground nutmeg
- 3 tablespoons butter
- 2 tablespoons grated Parmesan cheese

Instructions

1   Heat the spinach in a saucepan with 1/2 cup of water, until completely thawed. Strain the spinach, reserving half the amount of liquid.

2   Crumble the matzo into a medium-size mixing bowl and pour the spinach and the remaining liquid over

them. Mix thoroughly until the matzo are softened. Add the Parmesan, eggs, salt, nutmeg and pepper.

3   Heat the margarine in a 12 inch skillet and add the spinach mixture. Cook on medium heat, uncovered for 5 minutes on each side. Sprinkle with grated Parmesan and serve immediately.

Prep Time: 20 Minutes

Cook Time: 60 Minutes

Servings: 14

Ingredients

- 2 ¼ cups all-purpose flour
- 1 tablespoon pumpkin pie spice
- teaspoons baking powder
- ½ teaspoon salt
- 2 eggs
- 2 cups white sugar
- (15 ounce) can pumpkin puree
- ½ cup vegetable oil
- 1 cup dried cranberries
- 1 cup chopped walnuts

Instructions

1   Preheat oven to 350 degrees F (175 degrees C). Grease and flour 2 9x5 inch loaf pans (or 4 mini loaf pans).

2   In a mixing bowl, combine flour, pumpkin pie spice, baking powder and salt.

3   Combine eggs, sugar, pumpkin and oil in small mixing bowl, beat until just blended. Stir the wet mixture into the dry with a wooden spoon until batter is just moistened. Fold the cranberries and walnuts into the batter. Spoon the batter into the prepared loaf pans.

4   Bake in preheated oven for 50 to 60 minutes. (If using mini loaf pans, begin checking bread after 25 minutes.)

Ingredients

- tablespoons sesame seeds
- 2 cups shredded carrots
- 1 Granny Smith apple, cored and shredded
- ½ cup chopped fresh parsley
- ¼ cup lemon juice
- 2 tablespoons apple cider vinegar
- 1 tablespoon white sugar
- 1 clove garlic, minced
- 1 teaspoon salt
- ½ teaspoon ground black pepper
- 2 tablespoons safflower oil

Instructions

1. Heat a skillet over medium heat; pour sesame seeds into the hot skillet. Cook, stirring often, until sesame seeds are lightly browned and fragrant, 3 to 5 minutes. Remove from heat.
2. Mix carrots, apple, toasted sesame seeds, and parsley together in a bowl.

3   Whisk lemon juice, vinegar, sugar, garlic, salt, and pepper together in a separate bowl; slowly drizzle safflower oil into lemon juice mixture while continuing to whisk. Pour dressing over carrot mixture; toss to coat.

Prep Time: 15 Minutes

Cook Time: 20 Minutes

Servings: 2

Ingredients

- 1 ½ tablespoons olive oil, divided
- 1 cup pearl (Israeli) couscous
- 1 ½ cups boiling water
- 1 shallot, sliced
- 1 bunch asparagus, cut into 1-inch pieces
- Salt and freshly ground black pepper to taste
- 1 lemon, zested and juiced

Instructions

1 Heat 1/2 tablespoon olive oil in a medium saucepan over medium heat; add Israeli couscous. Toast couscous until lightly browned, 4 to 5 minutes. Slowly pour in boiling water. Cover and reduce heat to medium-low; simmer until couscous is tender and water has been absorbed, about 10 minutes.

2 Meanwhile, heat remaining olive oil in a large frying pan over medium heat. Add shallot and cook until starting to soften, about 1 minute. Increase heat to medium-high. Add asparagus and a pinch of salt; saute until asparagus is tender, 5 to 10 minutes.

3 Stir lemon zest into the asparagus in the last few minutes of cooking. Add cooked couscous and toss with the asparagus mixture. Stir in lemon juice. Taste for seasoning and add salt and pepper if needed.

Prep Time: 15 Minutes

Cook Time: 8 Minutes

Servings: 4

Ingredients

- tablespoons olive oil
- 2 cloves garlic, minced
- (14.5 ounce) can diced tomatoes
- tablespoons white wine
- 1 teaspoon dried sage
- 1 teaspoon dried thyme
- (15 ounce) can cannellini beans, drained and rinsed
- tablespoons chopped fresh basil
- Salt and pepper to taste
- cups arugula
- ¼ cup shaved Parmesan cheese (Optional)

Instructions

1   Heat the olive oil in a large skillet over medium heat; cook the garlic in the hot oil about 1 minute. Add the

tomatoes, wine, sage, and thyme; increase the heat to medium-high and simmer 2 to 3 minutes. Stir in the cannellini beans and basil. Season with salt and pepper. Continue cooking until beans are heated through, 3 to 4 minutes.

2 Arrange the arugula on a serving platter. Spoon the bean mixture over the arugula. Top with the shaved Parmesan cheese if desired.

Prep Time: 10 Minutes

Cook Time: 20 Minutes

Servings: 4

Ingredients

- ½ cup water
- ½ cup thinly sliced carrots
- ¼ cup red quinoa
- ½ teaspoon chicken bouillon granules
- 1 cup chopped cooked broccoli
- 1 cup baby spinach, chopped

Instructions

1 Combine water, carrots, quinoa, and chicken bouillon in a medium saucepan over medium heat. Bring to a boil; reduce heat and simmer until nearly all water has been absorbed and outer ring of quinoa grain is visible, 10 to 12 minutes.

2 Add broccoli and spinach to the pot, stir, and cover to allow spinach to wilt. Continue to cook until all water

is absorbed and vegetables have been heated through, about 5 minutes more.

3   Spoon quinoa and veggies into a bowl and serve.

Prep Time: 15 Minutes

Cook Time: 45 Minutes

Servings: 4

Ingredients

- (4 ounce) cube steaks
- medium potatoes, thinly sliced
- 1 large onion, thinly sliced
- teaspoons margarine
- Salt and pepper to taste

Instructions

1 Preheat the oven to 350 degrees F (175 degrees C).
2 Lay out 4 squares of aluminum foil. Place one cube steak onto each piece of foil. Spread margarine over the steaks, and season with salt and pepper. Layer one sliced potato over each steak, and a few rings of onion. Season again with salt and pepper if you like. Fold the foil around the food, and seal into a packet. Place packets onto a baking sheet.

3   Bake for 45 minutes in the preheated oven, until the beef is no longer pink, and the potatoes are tender. Open carefully, as hot steam will be released.

DINNERS

Prep Time: 10 Minutes

Cook Time: 35 Minutes

Total: 45 Minutes

Servings: 4

Ingredients

Vegetables:

- 1 tablespoon olive oil
- ½ teaspoon Greek seasoning (such as Cavender's®)
- 1 medium zucchini, cut in half and sliced
- 1 medium yellow squash, sliced
- ounces portobello mushrooms, quartered
- ounces fresh green beans, trimmed and halved
- 1 clove garlic, minced

Fish:

- ¼ cup pecans
- ¼ cup panko bread crumbs

- ½ teaspoon Greek seasoning (such as Cavender's®)
- 1 pound steelhead trout fillets
- 1 tablespoon melted butter

Rice:

- 1 (8.8 ounce) package long grain and wild rice (such as Uncle Ben's(R))
- 1 tablespoon water

Instructions

1 Preheat the oven to 425 degrees F (220 degrees C). Line a baking sheet with aluminum foil and spray with nonstick spray.

2 Combine olive oil and Greek seasoning in a bowl. Add zucchini, squash, mushrooms, green beans, and garlic, and toss to coat. Spread into a single layer on the prepared baking sheet.

3 Bake in the preheated oven for 10 minutes.

4 Meanwhile, prepare the crust for the fish. Place pecans in a high-frequency blender (such as Vitamix) and blend on high for 20 seconds. Transfer to a small bowl and mix in panko and Greek seasoning; set aside.

5   Remove vegetables from the oven and push them to one side of the sheet. Open the rice packet and carefully spread rice out on the empty side of the pan. Drizzle rice with water. Place trout fillets on top of the vegetables and rice. Brush fillets with melted butter and press panko mixture lightly into the fillets.

6   Bake in the preheated oven until fish easily flakes with a fork, about 20 minutes. Serve immediately.

Prep Time: 30 Minutes

Cook Time: 30 Minutes

Servings: 6

Ingredients

- medium shallots, halved, divided
- 1 cup baby arugula
- ½ cup loosely packed fresh mint leaves
- ½ cup loosely packed flat-leaf parsley
- tablespoons olive oil, divided
- teaspoons kosher salt, divided
- ¾ teaspoon ground black pepper, divided
- (1 1/2) pounds rack of lamb, trimmed and frenched
- 1 ½ pounds fingerling potatoes, halved lengthwise
- 1 pound tri-colored baby carrots
- 2 tablespoons red wine vinegar
- ¼ teaspoon crushed red pepper

Instructions

1   Place 2 shallot halves in a mini food processor. Pulse
    until coarsely chopped, about three 1-second pulses.
    Add arugula, mint, and parsley; pulse until herbs are
    chopped, about five 1-second pulses. Transfer 1/2 of
    the herb mixture to a small bowl. Reserve remaining
    herb mixture for serving.

2   Stir 4 tablespoons olive oil, 1 1/2 teaspoons salt, and
    1/4 teaspoon black pepper into the bowl with the herb
    mixture; rub all over meaty parts of lamb. Prop the
    two lamb racks up together on a plate by placing the
    meaty ends on the surface with the bones upright,
    interlacing the bones so they rest against each other.
    Let sit at room temperature for 1 hour.

3   Preheat the oven to 450 degrees F (230 degrees C)
    with racks in the upper and lower thirds. Line two
    large rimmed baking sheets with aluminum foil.

4   Meanwhile, toss potatoes, carrots, and remaining
    shallot halves with 2 tablespoons olive oil, 1 teaspoon
    salt, and remaining 1/2 teaspoon black pepper in a
    large bowl. Arrange in an even layer on the prepared
    baking sheets.

5   Roast vegetables in the preheated oven until
    beginning to brown and almost tender, about 15

minutes. Remove from the oven and combine onto one baking sheet. Set aside until ready to use. Do not turn the oven off.

6   Once lamb has marinated, place lamb racks onto the empty baking sheet.

7   Roast in the preheated oven for 10 minutes. Rotate the pan, scatter the roasted vegetables around the lamb, and continue to cook until a thermometer inserted into the thickest part of the lamb reads 125 degrees F (52 degrees C), 10 to 15 minutes longer. Remove from the oven and let rest for 10 minutes before slicing.

8   Stir remaining 3 tablespoons olive oil, vinegar, red pepper, and remaining 1/2 teaspoon salt into the reserved herb mixture. Drizzle over lamb and vegetables.

Prep Time: 30 Minutes

Cook Time: 35 Minutes

Servings: 8

Ingredients

- 1 (1.5 pound) head green cabbage
- 1 ½ pounds baby red potatoes
- tablespoons olive oil, divided
- teaspoons kosher salt, divided
- 1 teaspoon ground black pepper, divided
- (6 inch) matzo sheets
- tablespoons chopped flat-leaf parsley, divided
- 1 teaspoon lemon zest
- 2 tablespoons Dijon mustard
- (2 pound) skin-on salmon fillet
- tablespoons sherry vinegar
- 1 teaspoon Dijon mustard
- large hard-cooked eggs, chopped
- 2 tablespoons chopped fresh chives
- 2 tablespoons chopped cornichons
- 2 tablespoons non-pareil capers, rinsed and drained

Instructions

1 Preheat oven to 425 degrees F (220 degrees C) with a rack in the upper third. Line a large rimmed baking sheet with aluminum foil. Cut cabbage into 1-inch wedges.

2 Toss potatoes with 1 tablespoon of olive oil, 3/4 teaspoon salt, and 1/4 teaspoon pepper. Arrange in an even layer on the prepared baking sheet. Intersperse cabbage wedges on the baking sheet and brush with 1 tablespoon oil.

3 Bake in the preheated oven until starting to brown, about 15 minutes.

4 Meanwhile, break matzo sheets into large pieces and place in a zip-top bag. Carefully pound with the flat end of a glass until coarsely crushed; this should yield 2/3 cup. Transfer to a medium bowl and stir in 4 tablespoons parsley, 2 tablespoons oil, and lemon zest.

5 Spread 2 tablespoons Dijon mustard evenly over the top side of the salmon and sprinkle evenly with 1 teaspoon salt and remaining 3/4 teaspoon pepper. Press matzo mixture onto the mustard.

6 Remove potatoes and cabbage from the oven. Stir potatoes and flip cabbage, then push both to the sides

to make space in the center. Place salmon in the center and return to the oven. Bake until matzo is golden brown, potatoes and cabbage are tender, and salmon flakes easily with a fork, about 20 minutes.

7 While salmon bakes, whisk vinegar, 1 teaspoon mustard, and remaining 3 tablespoons oil together in a medium bowl. Fold in eggs, remaining 2 tablespoons parsley, chives, cornichons, capers, and remaining 1/4 teaspoon salt. Serve over salmon and vegetables.

Prep Time: 20 Minutes

Cook Time: 15 Minutes

Servings: 18

Ingredients

- ¾ cup pumpkin puree
- ¼ cup warm water
- ⅓ cup warm milk
- 1 large egg
- 1 tablespoon vegetable oil
- ¼ cups bread flour
- ¼ cup brown sugar
- 1 teaspoon salt
- 1 teaspoon pumpkin pie spice
- ¼ teaspoons quick-rising yeast

Instructions

1   Place pumpkin, water, milk, egg, oil, flour, sugar, salt, pumpkin pie spice, and yeast into a bread machine

pan in the order suggested by the manufacturer. Select Dough setting and press Start.

2   Turn dough out onto a lightly floured work surface. Shape into dinner rolls and place on lightly greased baking sheets. Cover with a towel and let rise until almost doubled in size, about 45 minutes.

3   Preheat the oven to 375 degrees F (190 degrees C).

4   Bake in the preheated oven until rolls are golden brown, about 15 minutes. Remove from the oven and immediately remove rolls from pans and cool on a wire rack to prevent crusts from becoming soggy.

Prep Time: 30 Minutes

Cook Time: 30 Minutes

Servings: 4

Ingredients

- 1 lemon, zested and juiced
- tablespoons olive oil
- 1 ½ teaspoons ras el hanout
- ½ teaspoon salt
- (6 ounce) bone-in chicken thighs with skin
- 1 medium sweet potato, peeled and cut into 1-inch chunks
- 1 medium zucchini, cut into 1-inch chunks
- (15 ounce) can chickpeas, drained and rinsed
- (14 ounce) can quartered artichoke hearts, drained
- 1 teaspoon ras el hanout
- ½ teaspoon salt
- tablespoons olive oil
- ¼ cup pomegranate seeds
- ¼ cup chopped fresh parsley
- tablespoons shelled pistachios, coarsely chopped

Instructions

1. Combine lemon juice, lemon zest, 2 tablespoons olive oil, 1 1/2 teaspoons ras el hanout, and 1/2 teaspoon salt in a resealable plastic bag. Place chicken thighs into the bag, making sure marinade gets under skin. Seal and refrigerate at least 30 minutes. Remove chicken from refrigerator 20 minutes before baking and let come to room temperature.

2. Preheat the oven to 400 degrees F (200 degrees C).

3. Combine sweet potato, zucchini, chickpeas and artichoke hearts in a bowl. Sprinkle with 1 teaspoon ras el hanout and 1/2 teaspoon salt. Drizzle with 2 tablespoons olive oil and stir to combine evenly.

4. Remove chicken from marinade and place on a 13x18-inch rimmed sheet pan. Place vegetable mixture around chicken.

5. Bake in the preheated oven, flipping vegetables halfway through, or until chicken has reached an internal temperature of 165 degrees F (74 degrees C), about 30 minutes.

6. Remove from oven and garnish with pomegranate seeds, parsley, and pistachios before serving.

Prep Time: 10 Minutes

Cook Time: 30 Minutes

Total: 40 Minutes

Servings: 6

Ingredients

- ½ pound dried elbow macaroni
- 1pound lean ground beef
- cloves garlic, pressed or minced
- medium carrots, quartered lengthwise and sliced
- 1 large zucchini, quartered lengthwise and sliced
- 1 ½ tablespoons dried oregano leaves
- Salt and pepper
- (10.75 ounce) can condensed tomato soup, plus
- (10.75 ounce) can water
- 1 ounce crumbled feta cheese

Instructions

1   Bring a large pot of lightly salted water to a boil. Cook
    elbow macaroni for 8 to 10 minutes or until al dente;
    drain, and set aside.

2   Brown ground beef with garlic in a large skillet over
    medium heat. Strain off fat, if necessary. When meat
    is lightly browned, add carrots and cook until tender,
    about 5 minutes. Stir in zucchini and oregano, and
    continue cooking another 5 minutes. Season to taste
    with salt and pepper.

3   When vegetables are tender, stir in tomato soup,
    water, and prepared elbow macaroni, and cook for
    another 5 to 10 minutes. Serve with crumbled feta
    cheese on top, if desired.

Prep Time: 20 Minutes

Cook Time: 30 Minutes

Servings: 6

Ingredients

- ¼ cup olive oil
- small zucchini, sliced
- small carrots, chopped
- 2 red bell peppers - cored, seeded, and cut into chunks
- 2 potatoes, peeled and cut into 1/2-inch cubes
- 15 cherry tomatoes
- 15 black olives
- green onions, chopped
- 2 cloves garlic, pressed or minced
- 2 teaspoons dried oregano, or to taste
- 2 teaspoons dried thyme, or to taste
- Salt and freshly ground black pepper to taste
- 2 sprigs rosemary
- 2 bay leaves
- 1 (4 ounce) package feta cheese, crumbled

Instructions

1. Preheat oven to 400 degrees F (200 degrees C). Grease 2 baking sheets with 2 tablespoons olive oil each.

2. Distribute zucchini, carrots, red bell peppers, potatoes, cherry tomatoes, black olives, and green onions between the 2 baking sheets. Season with garlic, oregano, thyme, salt, and pepper. Place 1 rosemary sprig and 1 bay leaf on each baking sheet.

3. Bake in the preheated oven until vegetables are lightly browned and easily pierced with a fork, 25 to 35 minutes. Remove from oven, distribute feta evenly between the 2 baking sheets, and return to oven. Bake until feta is slightly melted, 5 to 10 minutes.

Prep Time: 15 Minutes

Cook Time: 55 Minutes

Servings: 6

Ingredients

- pounds smoked pork shoulder
- Salt and pepper to taste
- large onions, quartered
- potatoes, peeled
- ounces carrots, cut in half
- 1 large head cabbage, quartered
- 1 pound fresh green beans, trimmed

Instructions

1. Place the smoked pork into a large pot and fill with enough water to cover. Season with salt and pepper, cover and bring to a boil. Reduce heat to low and simmer for about 30 minutes.

2. Add the carrots, potato, cabbage and onions; cover and continue to simmer. Use kitchen string to tie the

green beans into a bundle. Add them to the pot, cover and continue to cook until the carrots and potatoes are tender, about 25 minutes.

3   To serve, remove pork to a serving dish. Arrange vegetables around it. Allow the pork to rest about 10 minutes before slicing.

Prep Time: 35 Minutes

Cook Time: 55 Minutes

Servings: 6

Ingredients

- 2 ¼ teaspoons active dry yeast
- 1 cup warm water (110 degrees F/45 degrees C)
- ¼ cup dry potato flakes
- tablespoons white sugar
- 1 teaspoon salt
- 1 egg
- tablespoons vegetable oil
- ¾ teaspoon onion powder
- 2 ¼ cups all-purpose flour

Instructions

1 In a large bowl, dissolve yeast in warm water. Add potato flakes, sugar, salt, egg, vegetable oil, onion powder, and 1cup of the flour. Beat until smooth. Stir

in remaining flour. Continue stirring until smooth, scraping batter from sides of bowl.

2   Cover and let dough rise in warm place until doubled, about 20 to 30 minutes.

3   Preheat oven to 400 degrees F (200 degrees C). Lightly grease 12 muffin cups.

4   Punch down dough. Spoon dough into 12 greased muffin cups, filling each half full. Let rise until batter reaches tops of cups, or about 20 minutes.

5   Bake in a preheated 400 degree F(200 degrees C) for 15 minutes. Serve immediately.

Prep Time: 30 Minutes

Cook Time: 35 Minutes

Servings: 6

Ingredients

- 1 head cauliflower, broken into florets
- 1 head broccoli, broken into florets
- medium potatoes, peeled and cubed
- large bell peppers (any color), chopped
- ½ cup baby carrots, or to taste
- ½ large onion, chopped
- 1 teaspoon garlic powder, or to taste
- 1 teaspoon dried parsley, or to taste
- 1 teaspoon dried cilantro, or to taste
- 1 teaspoon dried Italian seasoning to taste
- Salt and freshly ground black pepper to taste
- 2 tablespoons olive oil, or as needed
- (12 ounce) package apple chicken sausage, thinly sliced and quartered
- (12 ounce) package Italian sausage, thinly sliced and quartered

Instructions

1. Preheat the oven to 400 degrees F (200 degrees C). Line 2 baking sheets with parchment paper.

2. Combine cauliflower, broccoli, potatoes, bell peppers, baby carrots, and onion in a large bowl. Season with garlic powder, parsley, cilantro, Italian seasoning, salt, and pepper. Add olive oil and both sausages; stir to combine. Spread out vegetables and sausage evenly on the prepared baking sheet. Season with more spices and olive oil if desired.

3. Bake in the preheated oven until vegetables are soft, 30 to 45 minutes.